I0423825

# THE
# GARLIC
# EFFECT

Discover the Powerful Health and Beauty
Benefits of Using Garlic You Never Knew
About

Sandi Lane

**Copyright © 2016  Sandi Lane**
All Rights Reserved. No part of this publication may be
reproduced in any form or by any means, including scanning,
photocopying, or otherwise without prior written permission of
the publisher or copyright owner.

**Limits of Liability, Disclaimer of Warranties & Terms of
Use**

This book is a general educational information product. As an
express condition to reading this book, you understand and
agree to following terms. The information and advice contained
in this book are not intended as a substitute for consulting with a
professional.

The publisher and author make no representations or warranties
with respect to the accuracy or completeness of the contents of
this work and specifically disclaim all warranties, including
without limitation warranties of fitness for a particular purpose.
No warranty may be created or extended by sales or promotional
materials. The advice and strategies contained herein may not be
suitable for every situation. This work is sold with the
understanding that the publisher is not engaged in rendering
legal, accounting, of the professional services. If professional
assistance is required, the services of a competent professional
person should be sought. Neither the publisher nor author shall
be liable for damages arising therefrom.

ISBN-10: 1533242801
ISBN-13: 978-1533242808

# DEDICATION

This book is dedicated to those in search of useful information on the many wonders of garlic and the proven benefits and preventions obtained through its natural use.

# CONTENTS

Introduction     i

1   GARLIC THROUGH THE YEARS   1

2   THE GARLIC EFFECT   5

3   GARLIC ON STUDY   21

4   ON GARLIC USE: SAFETY AND   25
PRECAUTIONS

# INTRODUCTION

Garlic, in some places, is considered a wonder drug with its many curative properties. It belongs to the onion family with relatives like onion, shallot and leek. A native of Central Asia and also frequently used in other parts of the world both for culinary and medicinal purposes

Garlic is effectively used in a plethora of natural treatments. Its medicinal value can be attributed to the presence of a sulphur-containing compound called 'allicin'. Allicin has anti-inflammatory, antibacterial, antiviral and antifungal properties. Garlic's health benefits are innumerable.

This book contains useful information on the many wonders of garlic and the proven benefits and preventions obtained through its natural use.

# CHAPTER 1 – GARLIC THROUGH THE YEARS

While these little bulbs are quietly stored inside your kitchens, let's take a quick travel to the past and discover the history of garlic.

In ancient times, the Greek offered piles of garlic as supper for the goddess Hecate while in ancient Egypt, these bulbs were worshipped as deities and inhabitants in some parts of the country even disliked the idea of garlic as food as it was sacred for them. Traditionally, garlic has been an amulet to ward off evil, especially in the early European and Chinese culture.

In Central Europe, garlic was hung in windows and rubbed onto chimneys and keyholes because it was believed to drive away demons, werewolves and vampires—a folkloric belief or superstition still depicted today in horror movies and books. Many cultures in Europe have also used garlic for protection or white magic. In other religions, however, such as Hinduism and

Jainism, garlic is believed to stimulate and warm the body and to increase an individual's desires; hence they avoid daily use of garlic, especially in preparation of food.

## Medicinal Purposes

Medicinally, even in the early years, garlic has already been used to prevent or treat a variety of diseases. Garlic was believed to be a natural healer. People all over the world had explored its uses, especially in the Far East. Traditional Chinese Medicine claims that the medicinal properties of garlic was first recorded as early as 2000 BCE wherein it accounts for the bulb's miraculous healing properties against poisoning. An anecdote tells us that there was one day when Yellow Emperor Huang-ti, while taking a walk with some companions, ate an aroid plant called yu-yu and was poisoned. He immediately ate a nearby plant and this cured him and his companions who also ate yu-yu. It turned out that the miraculous plant was garlic. Because of this incident, garlic earned a spot in the Chinese Herbal Medicine Materia Medica.

Besides traditional Chinese Medicine, garlic has also been one of the most widely used herbs in Ayurvedic medicine and traditional European medicine. In Indian Ayurveda, aside from its popular culinary use as a seasoning or condiment, garlic was also found to be one of the most effective antimicrobial herbs with activity against bacteria, fungi, and virus. Another popular Ayurvedic use was for gastric disturbances. As for traditional European use of garlic, it was recommended as a fumigant to aid release of the placenta. Garlic was also used for running sores and asthma. Hippocrates, Galen, Pliny the Elder, and Dioscorides, all big names of early medicine, have also cited garlic's beneficial effects in respiratory problems, poor digestion, low energy and its activity against parasites.

While garlic has become a very popular herb often used

for its flavoring properties in food preparations, its medicinal use is still trusted by many people. With the continuous innovation of instruments and methods, studies and research have found basis and support for the many known traditional medicinal uses of garlic. Some of garlic's unproven myths before have actually become a convenient truth for us today. Discover more on the power of this bulb as we go along.

## What's Inside That Bulb Anyway?

Belonging to the same family as onion, garlic is also known as Allium sativum L. It has long, narrow leaves which are flat like those of grass and an edible bulb containing cloves which are grouped together and enclosed by a whitish skin. The plant's bulb, which is the most utilized, holds the chemical constituents responsible for the many medicinal uses of garlic.

Garlic has approximately 33 sulfur compounds including alliin, allicin, and ajoene. Apart from these, garlic contains 17 amino acids and several enzymes and minerals. Nevertheless, the most important compound, alliin, an odorless sulfur compound, is converted to allicin when the bulbs are crushed. This allicin is responsible for the strong odor of garlic. It is, however, further broken down to ajoene to which the bulb's inhibitory action to blockage in blood vessels may be attributed.

Sandi Lane

# CHAPTER 2 – THE GARLIC EFFECT

Discover 14 surprising health and beauty benefits from garlic. That remedy you've been looking for may just be right inside your kitchen.

## (1)    A Natural Cardio-protective

Cardiovascular diseases remain as the leading cause of mortality worldwide. Among the major risk factors for these diseases are high blood pressure or hypertension and high cholesterol levels. To aid conventional medications, which often target management of blood pressure and cholesterol levels, some non-pharmacologic approaches using traditional and herbal medicine were found to be of significant value.

Many studies have proven garlic's role in the prevention and management of cardiovascular diseases. Blood pressure lowering, cholesterol level lowering, and blood-thinning activities related to it were found. Some researchers attribute the cardio-protective property of garlic to hydrogen sulfide, a gas generated from freshly crushed garlic. Hydrogen sulfide may be toxic in excess amounts but is beneficial to the heart in small but ample quantities. Because this gas is volatile and disappears as garlic is dried, processed, or cooked, researchers suggest intake of raw garlic cloves. Moreover, fresh garlic showed significantly greater effect in restoring blood flow in the aorta.

Chemical constituents found in fresh garlic may also be effective in keeping low density lipoproteins (LDL) or bad cholesterol level in a normal and healthy level thereby avoiding development of cardiovascular diseases. In a study published in the "Journal of Postgraduate Medicine" in 1991, a significant lowering of cholesterol levels in medical students who ingested a certain amount of garlic every day for a period of two months was documented. In another study, published in the "Pakistan Journal of Pharmaceutical Sciences" in 2006, it was found that consumption of raw garlic increased high density lipoprotein (HDL) levels and decreased total cholesterol.

Studies have also shown blood pressure lowering effect of garlic up to 5%-8%. It may slow down atherosclerosis or the hardening of arteries with age, as well. Garlic, as blood-thinner, may also suppress aggregation of blood platelets, thereby reducing risk for stroke and heart attack.

Today, supplements containing garlic extracts in the form of tablets and capsules are widely available in the market. Since these products, relatively, have more concentrated amount of the extract than raw garlic, some experts say these show more significant results. Nevertheless, consumption of the raw cloves is still advised by many for adjunctive purposes to current conventional medications being taken.

Eating a fresh clove of garlic, which approximately contains 1% alliin, a day is one way to get its heart-healthy benefits. Another way is to mince a clove, let it stand for 10-15 minutes, then mix with yogurt, applesauce, honey or any other vehicle.

## (2) Anti-inflammatory Agent

The significant anti-inflammatory property of garlic is attributed to its sulfur-containing compounds, ajoene, diallyl sulfide and thiacremonone. These chemicals have the ability to inhibit the production of pro-inflammatory mediators in the body. Now, garlic is being used in the management of arthritis and airway inflammation in allergic rhinitis. It was found helpful in alleviating the pain and swelling associated to rheumatoid arthritis. However, its potency significantly diminished after exposing garlic to heat; hence fresh cloves are recommended.

For management of allergic rhinitis, some homemade preparations are given below:

### Garlic tea

Add 4-5 cloves of minced or crushed garlic, fresh lemon juice and raw, unprocessed honey to four cups of boiled water which was cooled slightly. Drink 3-4 cups of this tea daily, either warm or cold. Remember not to re-boil the solution.

### Honey garlic syrup

On a tablespoon, place ½-1 crushed garlic clove and pour raw, unprocessed honey. Take a spoonful of this preparation every 4-6 hours as needed.

Lastly, raw garlic juice can be taken to ease itching due to rashes and bug bites.

## (3) Insect Repellent

More than driving werewolves and vampires away from your doors, garlic can protect you from some other things which can cause more harm. The strong pungent odor of garlic is found unpleasant by insects and masks the fragrance of their host plant which attracts them to it. This makes garlic effective for small sucking insects such as aphids and mosquitoes. Because of their soft bodies, they are more easily susceptible to the powerful stinging sensation caused by garlic. Gardeners often plant garlic to avoid insect pests to thrive. While a concentrated garlic spray can be prepared to kill pests, it can also be diluted to practically cover more area. Here are some ways to prepare garlic spray for your garden.

Recipe #1

Ingredients: finely crushed garlic (500 g), liquid paraffin (150-200 mL), pure soap (150 g), water (2.5 L)

Preparation: Macerate the garlic in adequate liquid paraffin for 24-48 hours. Add the remaining ingredients into the previous mixture and stir thoroughly. Filter the resulting mixture well using a commercial sieve or a piece of muslin cloth. Dilute the 15-20 mL of the concentrated filtrate with 1 L of water, depending on the desired use.

Recipe #2

Ingredients: chopped or crushed garlic (3-4 bulbs, approximately 100 g), mineral oil (40 mL), pure soap flakes (25 g), water (500 mL)

Preparation: Mix the chopped or crushed garlic with mineral oil, soap flakes and water and let the mixture stand for at least 24 hours. Filter the mixture and dilute every 15 mL of the concentrated filtrate with 1L of water.

The insect repellent effect of homemade garlic spray preparations usually lasts for 24-72 hours, depending on the temperature, moisture, and amount of direct sunlight in the environment.

As for human use, there are garlic-based insecticide and repellent preparations available commercially which are already proven effective against mites and mosquitoes. A homemade preparation may be made by mixing garlic oil, petroleum jelly and beeswax. This has to be applied to the skin like the other commercially available topical preparations.

## (4) The Anti-Athlete's Foot

True enough, you do not have to be an athlete to get this on your feet. Athlete's foot or scientifically, Tinea pedis, is a fungal infection which can be easily contracted from wet places such as gym locker rooms, swimming pools, and nail salons. It commonly effects active people, the elderly, and those who may have had it already before. People infected with athlete's foot experience a terribly discomforting and irritating sensation of itching, burning, and scaling of the skin. Most of the time, blisters appear between the toes, as well.

But no need to worry that much, 'cause your very own kitchen buddy is here again to save the day. For many years, garlic has been known as a powerful natural antifungal and this property is attributed to one of its chemical constituents, ajoene which is the end-product of further breaking down allicin from alliin.

Use of garlic solution for athlete's foot showed 100% cure when tested against a commercially available preparation which yielded only a 94% cure. Various antifungal creams and gels are available in the market. But with the infection's habit of returning after symptoms have subsided, it just causes an additional pain in the pocket. Nevertheless, garlic could be much cheaper and could even be free and just a backyard away.

To manage athlete's foot, prepare a basin of water with crushed garlic and soak your feet into the preparation for 30 minutes. Another option is to prepare a mixture of garlic and olive oil and apply this directly on the affected areas using cotton swab.

## (5) Hair Loss Solution

Both a health and beauty benefit, garlic is also effective in treatment of hair loss. Aside from the phytochemicals it contains, garlic stores minerals and vitamins which are essential to having healthy hair, as well. Among these hair-nourishing constituents are:

Copper

This mineral is very important in healthy hair growth. Since it is not produced by the body, adequate intake of copper-rich food such as garlic would help prevent hair loss and allow growth of thick hair. Copper is also associated to hair color intensifying benefits and prevention of graying of hair.

### Zinc

Another mineral found in garlic, zinc plays a vital role in the production of hair cells, as well. Moreover, zinc ensures a balance of copper levels to avoid copper-associated toxicities.

### Sulfur

Found abundantly in garlic, sulfur can increase blood circulation to the scalp thereby making it healthy and in turn stimulating hair growth. In the body, sulfur is needed in the hair, nails, and skin; hence deficiency in sulfur is often manifested by hair loss, brittle hair and nails, and dry skin.

### Vitamin C

Also known as ascorbic acid, vitamin C protects hair from breaking and helps boost collagen.

### Iron

This element provides nourishment in hair by carrying oxygen to hair follicles. In fact, one of the most common causes of hair loss in pre-menopausal women is iron deficiency.

While consumption of garlic as food is already helpful in the management of hair loss, topical application of a garlic preparation is another option. A home remedy is to crush garlic cloves and mix it with one teaspoon of coconut oil. Boil the mixture for a few minutes and stir gently then, allow it to cool. Apply the mixture to scalp in a gently massaging manner. Best results can be obtained by repeating this method two to three times a week.

Garlic is really your ultimate health solution from the toes to the head.

## (6) The Acne Remedy

Acne has always been a hindrance to beauty. Surprisingly, garlic could also be a remedy. Due to its antioxidant and antibacterial properties, garlic can help clear acne and banish blemishes. This effect can be achieved either by using garlic topically or ingesting it. Here are four ways on how to fight acne with garlic.

#1

Apply some pressure on a cut piece of fresh garlic to extract some juice. Then, rub this small piece onto the affected area. Leave it for five minutes then wash with cold water. Effect can be observed as reduction in redness and swelling within the day. This method also helps to prevent marks left by acne.

#2

If the previous method causes stinging on the skin, peel and crush some garlic cloves and add a teaspoon of honey and 2 teaspoons of yogurt, instead. Apply this as mask all over the face, and then wash within 20 minutes. Alternatively, garlic oil (not more than 2-3 drops), or garlic powder (not more than a half teaspoon) may be used.

#3

Another less stinging and burning method is to crush a clove of garlic and make a paste with a half cup of warm water. Apply this to face with a washcloth and then wash with a gentle cleanser. (Methods #2 and #3 should not cause irritation to the skin, otherwise, discontinue use).

#4

Take two cloves of fresh garlic with warm water regularly in the morning to reduce acne and give a glow to the skin.

## (7) The Total Anti-Aging Agent

Garlic contains several pharmacologically active components that boost the immune system generally improving one's health and help one fight diseases ranging from the less serious cough and colds to as serious as those associated to mortality. Garlic prevents one from acquiring serious health diseases. As mentioned in a previous section, components of garlic can prevent the development of heart diseases. It slows down atherosclerosis meaning, it can preserve the elasticity of blood vessels thereby decreasing the risk of having stroke. It also prevents accumulation of cholesterol deposits in vascular walls. Moreover, garlic reduces risk and may, as well, slow or stop growth of prostate and bladder cancers. It can also reduce development of digestive tract tumors.

Aside from keeping one healthy from within, garlic helps to keep a youthful outside radiance. Upon exposure to the sun's ultraviolet rays, the body forms metalloproteinases. These are enzymes that break down connective tissues which eventually lead to forming wrinkles and fine lines. The strong antioxidants in garlic, on the other hand, inhibit this free radical activity. Among the helpful antioxidants found in garlic are the minerals zinc and selenium, and vitamin C which is very much recognized for its ability to scavenge wrinkle causing free radicals. Sulfur in garlic also prevents wrinkles by helping the body produce collagen. Furthermore, garlic polyphenols, which protect the skin.

Garlic, therefore, keeps you young inside and out.

## (8) Relief of Toothache

A toothache can be felt as a mild soreness or it can be

an extremely painful sensation in the teeth and around the jaws. This develops when the part of a tooth called pulp becomes irritated or inflamed and one major cause is an infection. With its antibacterial action, many have found relief by using garlic. It is an effective palliative remedy to ease the pain until you can see a dentist.

It can be done by mixing a crushed garlic clove or some garlic powder with a pinch of table salt. This is applied to the affected tooth. Chewing one or two cloves of garlic can also work, alternatively.

## (9) The Healthy Weight Loss Buddy

It was discovered that garlic helps in burning more calories when supplemented to your daily activities. It also decreases the body's production of fats. A study in mice which were fed with a high-fat diet for eight weeks showed a reduction in their body weight and fat stores after supplementing the same diet with 2% to 5% garlic for the next seven weeks. Also, another study published in the journal "Nutrition Research and Practice" in 2012 obtained results that taking garlic extract every day for 12 weeks helped women lose weight and reduce their body mass index.

Though the exact explanation for garlic's weight loss power is still unclear, these are some hypotheses made by researchers. First is that allicin in garlic has an appetite suppressant property such that when garlic is eaten, it sends signals to the brain which tells you that you are already full. Another is that garlic increases metabolism which in turn helps burn calories and lose weight. Whichever is the reason, you might want to add garlic in your regular diet. Just let crushed fresh garlic sit at room temperature for 10 minutes before you use it in cooking. Of course, with proper diet and exercise, results would be better.

## (10) Treatment of Cold Sores

Well, this is both of a health and beauty concern. Cold sores are actually caused by the Herpes Simplex Virus (HSV) Type 1. These are blister-like lesions which appear anywhere in the body from two to twenty days after exposure to the virus. However, it most commonly manifests around the lips, nose, and chin. It is also, most of the time, accompanied by a tingling and stinging sensation. If left untreated, it generally spreads over the next two to three days. It is also very contagious when it is open.

Because these little bumps are very unsightly and embarrassing, you would most probably be very self-conscious and lose some self-esteem. Nevertheless, a very easy way to ward this off is by using garlic.

Garlic has excellent antiviral properties that make it effective for treating cold sores. For this purpose, you may eat the fresh raw clove or take the commercially available garlic supplements. Another safe way is to crush or scrape a garlic clove then add a few drops of olive oil and apply this on the affected area. Do this regularly until you observe your cold sores shrink and finally disappear.

Until full recovery, direct contact with other people should be avoided. Sharing of things such as razors, utensils, towels, and cups and kissing could easily spread the virus and lead to a breakout. Once the cold sores dry up and the crust goes away, then you are no longer contagious. However, the virus could come back and attack your body again if your immune system drops. Cold sores can actually develop due to some factors like colds and emotional and physical stress.

### (11) Dandruff No More

Having problems with an itchy scalp or white flakes falling off to your clothes? Worry no more; garlic is here to save the day again.

Garlic is proven to be an excellent natural remedy for dandruff, a common problem affecting both the young and the old all over the world. Dandruff is usually seasonal and occurs most during the winter when it is driest. It is commonly caused by dry skin, infrequent shampooing, seborrheic dermatitis, or infection by Malassezia, a fungus that naturally lives on the scalp of many adults. However, in some cases, it irritates the scalp. This irritation triggers more skin cells to grow. The extra skin cells then die and fall off.

Garlic can either be an oral or topical remedy for dandruff. Crushed garlic is highly packed with allicin, a natural antifungal. Simply spice up any dish with some crushed fresh garlic, which sat for about to 10 to 15 minutes. Alternatively, you can press some coconut and garlic using a piece of cloth and apply the filtered juice on the scalp for about half an hour then wash your hair afterwards.

### (12) Prevention of food poisoning

Diallyl sulfide, a chemical constituent of garlic, was found to be more effective than ciprofloxacin and erythromycin in fighting a leading cause of food poisoning,

Campylobacter sp. This compound, compared to the two antibiotics mentioned, can easily penetrate the slimy protective biofilm in Campylobacter organisms, which make them hard to destroy. By this mechanism, the bacterial cells are killed by shutting down their growth and metabolism.

Campylobacter sp. is said to be the most common bacterial cause of food-borne illness in the United States and the United Kingdom. Infections from this bacterial organism are usually acquired from eating raw or undercooked poultry or food that has been contaminated. In the UK, it was reported that Campylobacter sp. was responsible for 88 deaths in England and Wales in 2009.

Other studies found that the antibacterial property of garlic, that is fresh, is also effective against other food poisoning agents like Escherichia coli, Staphylococcus aureus, and Salmonella enteritidis.

## (13) Strep Throat Relief

Sore and scratchy throat? You might be experiencing strep throat. This is a bacterial throat infection caused by Streptococcus pyogenes. Although only a small portion of sore throats is actually strep throat, it is a highly contagious infection and can be spread by coughing or sneezing, or sharing food and drinks through airborne droplets. Strep throat causes a painful, itchy throat, and is often manifested with fever. Other symptoms include dysphagia or difficulty in swallowing, swollen tonsils and lymph nodes in the neck, and red spots on the soft or hard palate. Untreated strep throat can further lead to worse conditions including kidney inflammation and rheumatic fever.

Having both anti-inflammatory and antibacterial activities, garlic may help get rid of strep throat. This can be achieved by following these simple steps: Boil 1 cup of water. Place into the water four cloves of garlic and boil for an additional minute. Then, reduce the heat and let it simmer for five minutes. While doing so, you may inhale the steam to kill germs thriving in the mucus in the nose to prevent them from reaching the throat. Strain the boiled preparation through a piece of cheesecloth into a mug, add a teaspoon of honey and stir. Drink this tea regularly until symptoms resolve.

## (14) A Magic for Warts and Corns

Here are other hindrances to ones aesthetics: warts and corns. Warts are caused by the human papilloma virus (HPV). These can appear on different parts of the body. Often, they are seen on the fingers, which are called common warts, and on the soles of the feet, which are called plantar warts. These can spread easily by direct contact with scratches or cuts in the skin. On the other hand, corns are thickened skin that appears as small collections. They are usually found on the soles or sides of the feet due to excessive pressure or friction with footwear, or aggressive athletic activity.

In one recent clinical study published in the "International Journal of Dermatology," it was found that a fat-soluble garlic extract caused 100% recovery in patients with warts and 80% recovery in patients with corns while an aqueous garlic extract was found to eliminate small warts after 30-40 days.

In the absence of these extracts, a simple home remedy with garlic is very easy to do. Just peel one clove of garlic and cut it into half. Gently rub the wart or corn with the cut side of the garlic and be sure to coat the wart or corn with garlic juice. After doing this for 1-2 minutes, fix the other half of the garlic clove onto the wart or corn using an athletic tape. Apply this natural garlic treatment every night, before going to bed, then remove it on waking up in the morning to allow the area to breathe. Repeat the process until you see that it resolves. Following this remedy, small warts or corns are expected to resolve completely within a week while larger ones may take some weeks.

Sandi Lane

# CHAPTER 3 – GARLIC ON STUDY

This section features two other possible benefits from garlic which are still the focus of several studies and research today.

Prevention of Cancer

There have been several studies on the possible preventive ability of garlic against certain types of cancer. Laboratory studies involving the use of cell cultures and animal subjects show that garlic may help reduce growth of tumor. In some studies using cell cultures, it was found that garlic can help induce apoptosis of cancer cells, or the process of natural death of cells. Other studies have also determined possible activity of garlic against Helicobacter pylori, which is believed to be the major cause of stomach cancer. Animal studies, on the other hand, showed that garlic may help protect against skin, liver, colon, and breast cancer.

Data on studies involving human subjects are also available. The correlation between increased consumption of garlic and reduced risk of cancers such as that of the breast stomach, esophagus, colon, and pancreas has been found in many population studies. Upon analysis of data across seven population studies, it was concluded that higher intake of raw and cooked garlic lowered the risk of stomach and colorectal cancer. Another study showed that in women, those who consumed the highest amount of garlic had a 50% lower risk of cancer of the distal colon than those who consumed the least.

Furthermore, a recently concluded population-based case-control study which was conducted among a Chinese population from 2003-2010 showed that there is also an association between intake of raw garlic and lung cancer suggesting that garlic has preventive action for this type of cancer. In the United States, on the other hand, a hospital research suggested that selenium in garlic may possess an anti-cancer property and another said that the organosulfur compounds in garlic may play a part in killing brain cancer cells. However, while there are a lot of population-based and observational studies strongly suggesting the preventive ability of garlic, there are still a few randomized clinical trials, whose results could be more reliable, that dwell on this topic. Therefore, further investigations would be more helpful.

## 1. A Potential Hypoglycemic

In a recent study in animals, it was found that high doses of raw garlic significantly reduced blood sugar levels. In relation to this, an earlier research, also involving animals, found that garlic may increase insulin secretion thereby lowering blood sugar hence it is assumed that garlic intake may be helpful for patients with Type 2 Diabetes. In fact, some experts say that moderate intake of garlic supplements, and raw or cooked garlic or garlic extract can benefit diabetic patients as these may help regulate blood glucose and stop or lower the effects of some diabetes complications.

Scientists have found that allyl propyl disulphide, allicin, and S-allyl cysteine sulfoxide, all found in garlic, could work by blocking the liver's inactivation of insulin thereby increasing the amount of insulin in the blood, making it more available. Nevertheless, as we wait for better evidences on the hypoglycemic power of garlic, it could still be helpful to have it in moderate amounts as it may lessen effects of complications such as heart disease and stroke, hypertension, and arteriosclerosis.

Sandi Lane

# CHAPTER 4- ON GARLIC USE:
# SAFETY AND PRECAUTIONS

Garlic, as a condiment or seasoning, is generally safe for everyone. However, for its medicinal purposes, there are some important points that need to be known first before taking any action.

While garlic poses no risk at all for many, there are a few, like Dracula maybe, who might be allergic to it and may experience skin rash from touching or eating garlic. For those without the allergy, frequent eating or ingesting large amounts of garlic could cause bad breath, as its strong and pungent odor lingers in the mouth. When applied topically as a concentrated paste, it may cause a burning sensation to the skin.

During pregnancy and lactation, garlic intake in normal dietary amounts is also safe. However, if taken in higher amounts, some chemical constituents of garlic can be transmitted into the breast milk and cause colic in infants. Garlic may also pose health risks in children when taken orally in large doses.

Due to its blood thinning property, garlic may increase the risk of bleeding. Therefore, it is not recommended to be used in large amounts by persons with hemophilia or other bleeding disorders. Patients who are scheduled for a surgery should stop taking garlic at least two weeks before the surgery as it may prolong bleeding. Intake of therapeutic amounts should be avoided, as well, during post-surgical care to allow wound healing. Patients who are on warfarin (Coumadin) medication should avoid large amounts of garlic, too, as it may amplify the anti-coagulation activity of warfarin and might cause the patient to experience bruising and bleeding.

Caution should also be taken by diabetic patients who are on insulin or oral anti-diabetic medications. Because garlic is suspected to have anti-hyperglycemic effect, it may cause blood glucose to drop when taken with such medications and may lead to hypoglycemia.

Garlic may also irritate the gastrointestinal tract so care should be taken if you have stomach or digestion problems.

Medicinal preparations of chopped garlic in oil should not be left to stand at room temperature for several hours to prevent growth of certain harmful bacteria.

Patients who are taking isoniazid, an anti-mycobacterial or anti-tuberculosis drug, should avoid intake of garlic as it disturbs absorption of the said drug. Garlic decreases the amount of isoniazid that the body absorbs thereby decreasing the drug's effect. Similarly, garlic interacts with HIV/AIDS medications called Non-Nucleoside Reverse Transcriptase Inhibitors (NNRTIs) by inducing the body's metabolism of these drugs causing them to be broken down more quickly and lessening their effectiveness. Among the NNRTIs are nevirapine, delavirdine, and efavirenz.

By learning about the possible side-effects and the known contraindications and drug interactions of garlic, one could be guided when planning to use it for its health and beauty purposes. Using garlic for a short period of time or for its quick-relief purposes might not be that of a problem. But if planning on taking it complimentarily with current medications, it is always best to consult a GP or any health practitioner

Once you've chosen your turmeric roots, there's two ways you can go about planting them. First, you can plant the whole thing. Just make sure you place the side that has the most buds upwards. The other method is to cut off the buds and plant them one by one.

Turmeric thrives in well-draining soil. Prepare your soil first by moistening it a bit so tilling will be a bit easier. You can likewise use garden pots or containers filled with soil. Dig two inch deep holes that are at least a foot apart. Afterwards, place a root in each hole with the buds facing upwards. If you're using pots, place them in an area that gets full sun. Turmeric likes the temperature to be somewhere between 20 to 30°C. You can transplant the sprouts later on to your garden if you wish.

Water them regularly but be careful not to overwater. Root rot is one of the major problems in growing turmeric and too much water will do just that. You'll notice sprouts after a few weeks but it will take around eight to ten months before you can start harvesting the roots.

### *Please Leave a Review*

Finally, if you enjoyed this book, please take the time to share your thoughts and post a review. It would be greatly appreciated.

That review and feedback will help me improve the content in my books – and make each and every one more relevant and helpful to you.

Thank you again and good luck!


Sandi Lane

www.ingramcontent.com/pod-product-compliance
Lightning Source LLC
Chambersburg PA
CBHW061929280526
45787CB00004B/1539

* 9 7 8 1 5 3 3 2 4 2 8 0 8 *